Cooking Ta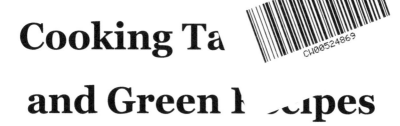
and Green l ⌐ipes

50 Mouthwatering

Homemade Meals to

Boost Weight Loss and

Kill Hunger

By

Spoons of happiness

Table of Contents

Introduction

A healthy lifestyle includes weight maintenance, continuous exercise and a healthy diet. All this will contribute to avoid health problems such as obesity, heart disease, diabetes, hypertension, among others. That is why the Lean and Green Diet is designed to help you achieve the goal of losing weight, maintain it over time, avoid the rebound effect, and help you improve your lifestyle.

The Lean and Green diet is designed to provide low calories and few carbohydrates to the body, increasing the intake of lean proteins and green vegetables, which will be used as a source of energy. In this regard, it is important to note that lean meats are obtained from poultry or fish and have less than 10% fat. Some examples are chicken, rabbit, veal and different varieties of fish.

The consumption of this type of meat is recommended in low-fat or high protein diets.

In addition to being high in protein, lean meats have properties such as being a good source of zinc, being sugar-free, high in iron, potassium, calcium, phosphorus, iodine, magnesium, sodium, vitamins and fiber, as well as being low in cholesterol and saturated fats.

Vegetables and green vegetables are an excellent source of nutrients for our health, since they provide the body with a variety of minerals, vitamins and fiber, which is why their consumption is essential in any balanced and healthy diet.

By combining the consumption of lean meats with green vegetables and little amount of balanced fats, with the Lean and Green diet, we obtain the result of a low calorie and low carbohydrate diet that has as main effect the slimming, because by reducing carbohydrates, decreases the level of insulin in the body, which causes the body to burn the accumulated fat to use as energy.

Now, the Lean and Green diet may be ideal for you for the following reasons:

- You want to lose weight or maintain your weight by limiting carbohydrate intake.
- You are looking to improve your eating habits completely
- You enjoy varied, low-carb foods.

So with this Lean and Green cookbook, we will accompany you on the road to weight loss so you can totally change your life.

Chapter 1: Snacks Recipes

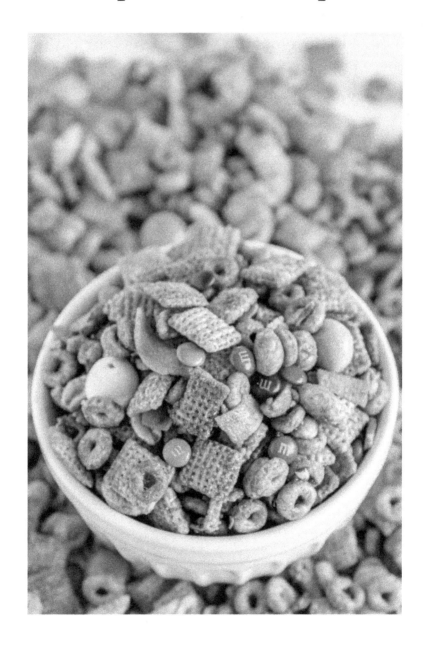

In this chapter, we are going to give you some delicious and mouthwatering recipes on Octavia Snacks recipes.

1. Caramel Snack Mix

(Ready in 1 Hour and 30 Minutes, Serve 20, Difficulty: Normal)

Nutrition per Serving:

Calories 226, Protein 3.4 g, Carbohydrates 36.9 g, Fat 12.6 g, Cholesterol 12.2mg, Sodium 182.6mg.

Ingredients:

- ½ cup of butter

- ¾ cup of white-corn syrup

- 1 cup of packed brown sugar

- 1 cup of chopped pecans

- 1 cup of almonds

- 1(12 ounces) package of crispy corn and rice cereal

Instructions:

1. Preheat the oven to 275 degrees Fahrenheit (135 degrees Celsius). Spray a large roasting pan with a non-stick cooking spray.

2. Mix the white corn syrup, butter, and brown sugar in a medium-sized, microwave-proof bowl. In a microwave, place the mixture and cook for 2 minutes, or until the butter melts.

3. In the prepared roasting pan, put the cereal, pecans, and almonds. Pour the molten butter mixture over the nuts and cereal and blend gently until the nuts and cereal are coated.

4. Bake for 1 hour, stirring every 15 minutes.

5. Since the snack mix is cooling, make sure to continue to mix so that the mixture will not harden in one big lump.

2. Clam Fritter Snacks

(Ready in 10 Minutes, Serve 4, Difficulty: Normal)

Nutrition per Serving:

Calories 230, Protein 21.6 g, Carbohydrates 22.2 g, Fat 14 g, Cholesterol 93.4mg, Sodium 473.8mg.

Ingredients:

- 1(10 ounces) can of minced clams, drained

- 1 cup of baking mix

- 1 egg, beaten

- 2 tablespoons of vegetable oil

Instructions:

1. Drain the clams. Beat one egg in a medium bowl and stir in the cup of baking mix and the clams.

2. Heat the oil in a medium skillet and fry the clams in pieces until they are golden brown.

3. drain them on a tray lined with paper towels.

3. Sweet Party Mix

(Ready in 1 Hour and 20 Minutes, Serve 2, Difficulty: Normal)

Nutrition per Serving:

Calories 267, Protein 3 g, Carbohydrates 35.6 g, Fat 13.9 g, Cholesterol 15.3mg, Sodium 176.6mg.

Ingredients:

- 1(12 ounces) package of crispy corn and rice cereal

- 5 ounces of slivered almonds

- 6 ounces of toasted, chopped pecans

- ¾ cup of butter

- ¾ cup of dark corn syrup

- 1 ½ cup of light brown sugar

Instructions:

1. Preheat the oven to 250 degrees Fahrenheit (120 degrees Celsius). Grease a large roasting pan lightly.

2. Mix the crispy corn and rice cereal, the slivered almonds, and the toasted, diced pecans in a large bowl.

3. Melt the butter and blend it with dark corn syrup and light brown sugar in a medium saucepan over medium heat.

4. Pour the mixture over the crispy corn and rice cereal mixture. Stir and shake to coat all the nuts and cereal.

5. In the prepared roasting pan, pour the covered mixture into it. Cook in the preheated oven for 1 hour, stirring evenly after 15 minutes.

6. Cool on wax paper and put in airtight containers.

4. No-Bake Energy Balls

(Ready in 35 Minutes, Serve 20, Difficulty: Normal)

Nutrition per Serving:

Calories 211, Protein 3.1 g, Carbohydrates 12.6 g, Fat 6.5 g, Cholesterol 0mg, Sodium 31.8mg.

Ingredients:

- 1 cup of old-fashioned oats

- ½ cup of peanut butter

- ½ cup of ground flax seed

- ½ cup of chocolate chips

- ⅓ cup of honey

- 1 tablespoon of chia seeds (Optional)

- 1 teaspoon of vanilla extract

Instructions:

1. In a cup, combine the oats, ground flax seeds, peanut butter, chocolate chips, sugar, chia seeds, and vanilla extract. Cover and cool the dough for 30 minutes in the refrigerator.

2. Remove the dough from the freezer, roll it into balls, around 1 inch in diameter.

5. Chex® Muddy Buddies

(Ready in 25 Minutes, Serve 18, Difficulty: Normal)

Nutrition per Serving:

Calories 206, Protein 3.2 g, Carbohydrates 30.7 g, Fat 9 g, Cholesterol 6.8mg, Sodium 192.2mg.

Ingredients:

- 9 cups of Rice Chex®, Corn Chex®, or Chocolate Chex® cereal (or combination)

- 1 cup of semisweet chocolate chips

- ½ cup of peanut butter

- ¼ cup of butter or margarine

- 1 teaspoon of vanilla

- 1 ½ cup of powdered sugar

Instructions:

1. Measure the cereal in a large bowl and put it aside.

2. Microwave peanut butter, chocolate chips, and butter uncovered on high for 1 minute, in 1-quart microwaveable bowl and stir.

3. Microwave for 30 seconds longer or before it is possible to smoothly stir the mixture. Stir in the vanilla Pour over the cereal mixture, stirring until evenly coated. Pour in a plastic container with 2-gallon resalable food-storage.

4. Add sugar powder. Shake until well coated. Seal the container. Spread to cool on waxed parchment.

5. Store in a refrigerator in airtight packages.

Chapter 2: Breakfast Recipes

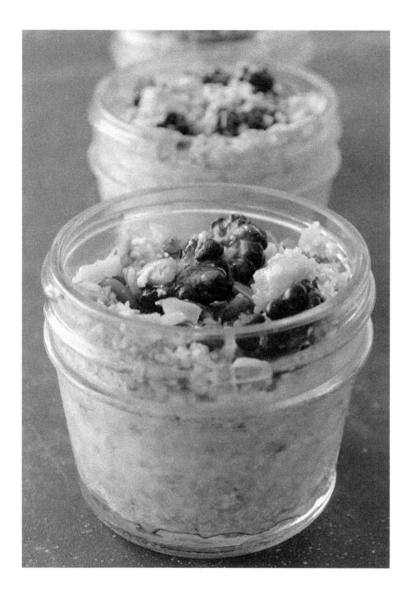

In this chapter, we are going to give you some delicious and mouthwatering recipes on Octavia Breakfast recipes.

1. No-Cook Overnight Oatmeal

(Ready in 8 Hours and 5 Minutes, Serve 4, and Difficulty: Easy)

Nutrition per Serving:

Calories 279, Protein 9.5 g, Carbohydrates 41.1 g, Fat 9.6 g, Cholesterol 17.8mg, Sodium 69.2mg.

Ingredients:

- ⅓ cup of milk

- ¼ cup of rolled oats

- ¼ cup of Greek yogurt

- 2 teaspoons of chia seeds

- 2 teaspoons of honey

- 1 teaspoon of ground cinnamon

- ¼ cup of fresh blueberries

Instructions:

1. In a 1/2-pint jar with a lid, mix milk, peas, Greek yogurt, chia seeds, sugar, cinnamon, cover, and shake until mixed.

2. Remove the cover and fold the blueberries together. Cover the jar with a cap.

3. Refrigerate the oatmeal overnight for 8 hours.

2. Muffin Pan Frittatas

(Ready in 35 Minutes, Serve 1, Difficulty: Normal)

Nutrition per Serving:

Calories 319, Protein 6.1 g, Carbohydrates 1.5 g, Fat 7 g, Cholesterol 103.7mg, Sodium 146.5mg.

Ingredients:

- Cooking spray

- 1 tablespoon of olive oil

- 1 cup of chopped fresh asparagus

- ¼ cup of chopped green bell pepper

- 2 tablespoons of chopped red onion

- 6 eggs

- ½ cup of milk

- ¼ teaspoon of salt

- ⅛ teaspoon of ground black pepper

- 1 cup of shredded cheddar cheese

Instructions:

1. In a medium-hot saucepan, heat the olive oil, cook and stir the asparagus, green bell pepper, and onion in the hot oil until softened, for 5-10 minutes.

2. In a bowl, combine the eggs, milk, salt, and black pepper. Mix the egg mixture with the cooked vegetables and cheddar cheese. Spoon a mixture of around ¼ cup into each muffin cup.

3. Bake in the preheated oven for about 20 minutes until the frittatas are set in the middle and lightly browned.

3. Chia Seed Pudding

(Ready in 10 Minutes, Serve 6, Difficulty: Normal)

Nutrition per Serving:

Calories 312, Protein 7.1 g, Carbohydrates 38.2 g, Fat 7.9 g, Cholesterol 1mg, Sodium 158.9mg.

Ingredients:

- 1 cup of unsweetened vanilla-flavored almond milk

- 1 cup of vanilla fat-free yogurt

- 2 tablespoons of pure maple syrup

- 1 teaspoon of pure vanilla extract

- ⅛ teaspoon of salt

- ¼ cup of chia seeds

- 1-pint of strawberries, hulled and chopped

- 4 teaspoons of pure maple syrup

- ¼ cup of toasted almonds

Instructions:

1. In a cup, whisk together almond milk, tofu, 2 teaspoons maple syrup, vanilla, and salt until combined, add chia seeds, whisk to combine, and let the chia seeds soak for 30 minutes.

2. To reallocate seeds that have settled throughout the mixture, stir the chia seed mixture. Cover the bowl with plastic wrap and chill overnight for 8 hours.

3. Sprinkle 4 teaspoons of maple syrup in a bowl over the strawberries, stir to cover. Add strawberries with almonds, stir.

4. Spoon the mixture of chia seeds into four containers, each with a part of the strawberry mixture.

4. Peanut Butter Banana Smoothie

(Ready in 5 Minutes, Serve 4, Difficulty: Easy)

Nutrition per Serving:

Calories 133, Protein 12.8 g, Carbohydrates 34.1 g, Fat 18.8 g, Cholesterol 9.8mg, Sodium 202.8mg.

Ingredients:

- 2 bananas, broken into chunks

- 2 cups of milk

- ½ cup of peanut butter

- 2 tablespoons of honey, or to taste

- 2 cups of ice cubes

Instructions:

Place the banana, peanut butter, honey, milk, and ice cubes in a blender and blend for about 30 seconds until smooth.

5. Yogurt Parfait

(Ready in 10 Minutes, Serve 1, Difficulty: Easy)

Nutrition per Serving:

Calories 121, Protein 21.4 g, Carbohydrates 68.2 g, Fat 17.8 g, Cholesterol 12.3mg, Sodium 177.1mg.

Ingredients:

- 2 cups of vanilla yogurt

- 1 cup of granola

- 8 blackberries

Instructions:

1. Layer 1 cup of yogurt, 1/2 cup of granola, and 4 blackberries into a big glass.

2. Place layers to repeat.

Chapter 3: Lunch Recipes

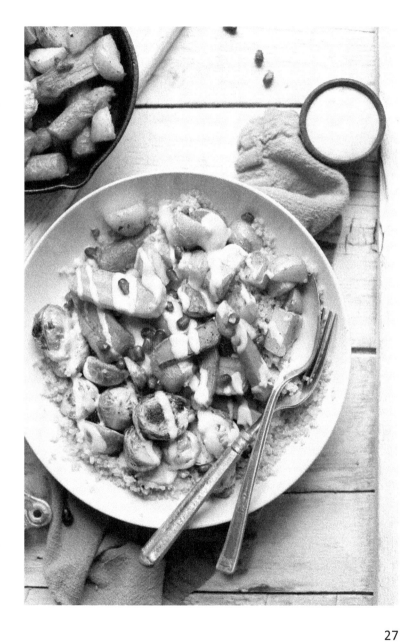

In this chapter, we are going to give you some delicious and mouthwatering recipes on Octavia Lunch recipes.

1. Easy Coconut Rice (South Indian Recipe)

(Ready in 35 Minutes, Serve 4, Difficulty: Easy)

Nutrition per Serving:

Calories 290, Protein: 5.4 g, Carbohydrate: 30 g, Fat 16.5 g, Fiber 4.2 g.

Ingredients:

- 2 tablespoons of oil

- ½ tablespoon of peanut

- 1 teaspoon of mustard seeds

- 1 teaspoon of cumin seeds

- ½ tablespoon of soaked chickpeas

- ½ tablespoon of soaked black gram

- 10 curry leaves

- 1 red whole chili

- ½ green chili

- 12 cashewnuts

- ½ teaspoon of salt

- 1 cup of grated coconut

- 2 cups of basmati rice (cooked)

- 2 tablespoons of grated coconut

Instructions:

1. Take a pan of oil and add the peanuts.

2. Add the mustard seeds to the peanut and cook them together, then add the cumin seeds and mix them, followed by the black gram and the soaked chana.

3. Cook all the ingredients together.

6. Now add the curry leaves, the whole red chili, and the chili green.

7. Cook them completely.

8. Add the cashew nuts to the pan, followed by salt, and combine well.

9. Now add to the pan the grated coconut.

10. To infuse the coconut flavor completely, combine the coconut thoroughly with the other ingredients.

11. Put the cooked rice in the pan now.

12. Mix them well.

13. To the rice, add grated coconut and mix again.

14. Serve it hot.

2. Flax Seed Raita (Indian Recipe)

(Ready in 25 Minutes, Serve 8, Difficulty: Easy)

Nutrition per Serving:

Calories 144, Protein 5.2 g, Carbohydrates 7.4 g, Fat 8.1 g, Cholesterol 16mg.

Ingredients:

- 3 tablespoons of flax ground seeds

- 1 cup of bottle grated gourd

- 1 cup of low-fat curd

- ½ cup of finely chopped, mint leaves

- 1 ½ teaspoon of coarsely ground, roasted cumin seeds

- Sal, to taste

- 1 cup of water

Instructions:

1. Combine water with the bottle guard. Cover and cook for 4 minutes on a medium flame.

2. Combine all the ingredients in a deep bowl, including the cooked gourd bottle, and blend well.

3. For at least 1 hour, refrigerate and serve chilled.

3. Oats Khichdi

(Ready in 30 Minutes, Serve 6, Difficulty: Easy)

Nutrition per Serving:

Calories 157, Protein 6.6 g, Carbohydrate 20.6 g, Fat 5.4 g, Fiber 3.1 g.

Ingredients:

- 1/3 cup of quick-cooking oats

- 1/3 cup of split skinned moong dal

- ½ teaspoon of cumin seeds

- ¼ teaspoon of turmeric powder

- ¼ tablespoon of red chili powder

- 1 small onion, finely chopped

- 1 medium tomato, finely chopped

- 1 small carrot, chopped

- 45 g of green peas

- ¾ teaspoon of finely chopped ginger

- ½ teaspoon of chopped green chilies

- 1 tablespoon of salt

- ½ tablespoon of extra virgin olive oil

- 2 cups of water

For Garnishing:

- ½ tablespoon of chopped fresh coriander leaves

Instructions:

1. In a pressure cooker, add oil, heat the oil, add cumin seeds and let them crackle.

2. Add the chopped onion and cook until translucent, add the ginger and green chilies, and cook for a few seconds.

3. Add the turmeric and red chili powder, then add the tomatoes. Let them cook until they're tender.

4. Add all vegetables and oats, along with rinsed moong dal. Cook for a couple of seconds.

5. Add water and adjust salt as per taste.

6. Cook for 8 minutes, through pressure.

7. Let the pressure calm down and open the lid.

8. Serve hot, served with yogurt, garnished with chopped coriander leaves or green chilies.

4. Curd Rice

(Ready in 25 Minutes, Serve 8, Difficulty: Easy)

Nutrition per Serving:

Calories 376, Protein 8.5 g, Carbohydrate 36.9 g, Fat 18.7 g, Fiber 1.8 g.

Ingredients:

- 1 cup of rice

- 3 cups of water

- 1 ½ cup of curd

- ½ cup of milk

- 1 carrot

- 1 green chili

- 1 teaspoon of ginger

- 1 teaspoon of salt

- 1 bunch of coriander leaves

- 2 teaspoon of oil

- 2 teaspoon of mustard seeds

- 1 teaspoon of chickpeas

- 2 teaspoon of black gram

- 2 bunch of curry leaves

- 2 red chili

- ½ teaspoon of hing

Instructions:

1. Add rice and water and cook it under pressure.

2. To make it soggy, mix the pressure-cooked rice a little bit.

3. Fill it with curd and milk and mix well.

4. Put the carrot, the green chili, the ginger, the salt, and the coriander's leaves. Thoroughly stir the ingredients.

5. Take a pan now, heat it, and pour in some oil.

6. To make a tadka, add mustard seeds, curry leaves, chickpeas, black gram, red chili, and hinges together.

7. Cook them thoroughly.

8. Place the curd rice in a bowl to serve and pour the tadka over it.

5. Spicy Curd Fry (Indian Recipe)

(Ready in 15 Minutes, Serve 2, Difficulty: Easy)

Nutrition per Serving:

Carbs 11 g, Protein 6 g, Fat 9 g, Fiber 2 g, Sugar 7 g, Sodium 25.4 g.

Ingredients:

- 1 onion, chopped

- 1 tomato, chopped

- 10-12 pieces of curry leaves

- ½ teaspoon of turmeric

- ½ teaspoon of salt

- ½ teaspoon of red chili powder

- 1 teaspoon of butter

- 1 bowl of chilled curd

Instructions:

1. Place some butter in a frying pan.

2. Add the onion and tomatoes and fry them together.

3. Stir in the turmeric, salt, and red chili pepper. Mix thoroughly.

4. Put the curry leaves together, mix well, and cook for a while.

5. The cooked tadka is added to the chilled curd.

6. Serve cold.

6. Baked Vegetables Casserole

(Ready in 30 Minutes, Serve 6, Difficulty: Easy)

Nutrition per Serving:

Calories 158.5, Protein 9.7 g, Fat 5.7 g, Cholesterol 5.9mg, Sodium 479.9mg,

Sugars 3.4 g.

Ingredients:

- 4 cups of vegetables (Your choice)

- 2 cups of cubed bread

- 1 cup of milk

- ¼ cup of butter milk

- 1 tablespoon of butter

- 1 teaspoon of olive oil

- 2 egg whites

- 1 bunch of rosemary

- 2-3 saga leaves

- Salt, to taste

- 1 teaspoon of chili peppers, roasted

Instructions:

1. Preheat the oven for 5 minutes at 140 degrees Celsius (284 F).

2. Grease an oven-proof dish with olive oil and toss butter with vegetables, bread, salt, and herbs to make them well coated.

3. Roast the vegetables at 180 degrees Celsius (356 F) for 15 minutes in the oven.

4. Combine the milk, butter, cheese, and eggs until the vegetables are roasted.

5. Take it out and pour in the milk and egg mixture after the vegetables are roasted and put it back in the oven.

6. Tear it into pieces if you are using cheese slices, then put it on top of the vegetables.

7. Cook for 15 minutes, until the mixture of milk and eggs is well cooked.

8. Serve it warm.

Chapter 4: Dinner Recipes

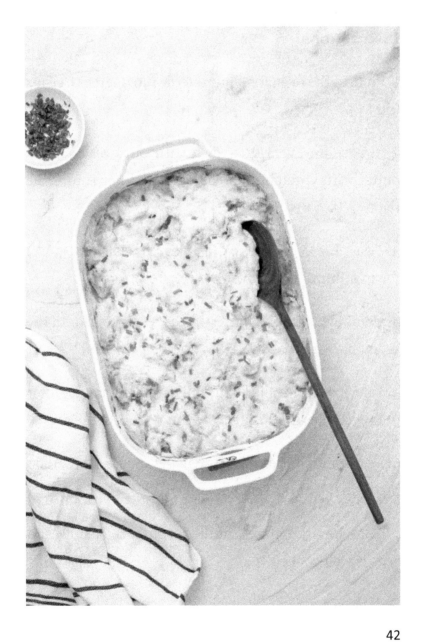

In this chapter, we are going to give you some delicious and mouthwatering recipes on Octavia Dinner recipes.

1. Chicken Cordon Bleu Casserole–Low Carb

(Ready in 45 Minutes, Serve 8, Difficulty: Normal)

Nutrition per Serving:

Calories 232, Protein 34 g, Carbohydrates 2 g, Fat 34 g, Sodium 916mg, Potassium 348mg, Sugar 1 g.

Ingredients:

- 6 cups of shredded cooked chicken (From about 2 pound of chicken)

- 6 ounces of ham cut into bite-size pieces

- 4 ounces of butter melted

- 6 ounces of softened cheese cream

- 1 tablespoon of Dijon mustard

- 1 tablespoon of white wine (optional)

- 1 ounces of lemon juice

- 1/2 teaspoon of salt

- 5 ounces of Swiss cheese

Instructions:

1. Preheat the oven to 350 degrees Fahrenheit (176 Celsius). Put the chicken in a 9x13-inch baking dish at the bottom of the pan. Layer the pieces on top of the ham.

2. Combine melted butter, white wine (if used), softened cream cheese, mustard, lemon juice, and salt in a large bowl with an electric mixer. Blend until it forms a thick sauce. In the baking dish, spread this sauce over the chicken and ham.

3. Place the Swiss cheese slices on top of the sauce. Bake until sweet, for 30-40 minutes.

4. At the end, I broiled it for 2 minutes so that the cheese will become bubblier and more golden. Do not leave it unattended if you have agreed to do so. The cheese topping is easy to burn.

2. Chili Pasta Bake

(Ready in 40 Minutes, Serve 6, Difficulty: Normal)

Nutrition per Serving:

Calories 102, Protein 29.5 g, Fat 25.5 g, Saturated Fat 12.6 g, Sodium 1248.3mg, Sugars 6.9 g.

Ingredients:

- 10 ounces of penne pasta

- 453 gramsof ground beef

- 1 medium onion, chopped

- 2 tablespoons of chili powder

- 1(14 1/2 ounces) can of canned tomatoes, diced cut

- 1(8 ounces) can of tomato sauce

- 1 cup of sauce

- 1(7 ounces) can of diced green chilies, drained

- 2 cups of shredded longhorn cheddar cheese

Instructions:

1. According to package instructions, prepare the pasta, drain.

2. Spray, set aside, a 13x9-inch pan with cooking spray.

3. Preheat the oven to 350 F (176 Celsius)..

4. In a large saucepan, cook the meat and onion and drain.

5. To the meat mixture, add the chili powder, tomato sauce, undrained tomatoes, salsa, and chilies.

6. Cook for five more minutes, add the cooked pasta to the mixture and mix well.

7. Pour into the prepared dish, top with the cheese, and bake for 20 minutes in a preheated oven or until thoroughly melted and bubbly.

3. Easy Burrito Bowl

(Ready in 25 Minutes, Serve 4, Difficulty: Normal)

Nutrition per Serving:

Calories 319, Protein 23.8 g, Carbohydrates 18.6 g, Fat 18.3 g, Sugar 1.8 g, Sodium 308 mg, Fiber 6.1 g.

Ingredients:

- 1 boneless, skinless chicken breast

- 2 cups of roughly chopped romaine lettuce

- ⅔ cup of cooked quinoa

- ½ avocado, sliced

- 1 lime

- 1 dash of chili powder

- ½ cup of cherry tomatoes, sliced in ½

- 4 tablespoon of low-fat shredded cheddar cheese

- Hot sauce (optional)

Instructions:

1. Sprinkle all sides of the chicken breast with chili powder.

2. Bake the chicken breast in the oven for 30-40 minutes at 400 degrees F (204 Celsius), until the chicken is fully cooked.

3. Slice it up into bite-sized chunks when the chicken is cooked.

4. Spread out 1/2 cup of quinoa, 1 cup of lettuce, and 1/4 cup of tomatoes to assemble each bowl.

5. To the cups, add the chicken, top with the avocado slices, and squeeze ½ lime of juice over each dish.

6. Finally, over each bowl, sprinkle 2 tablespoons of cheese and add hot sauce, if desired.

4. White Beans With Spinach and Sausage

(Ready in 35 Minutes, Serve 6, Difficulty: Normal)

Nutrition per Serving:

Calories 230, Protein 14 g, Carbohydrate 20 g, Fat 9 g, Fiber 6 g, Sodium 890 mg.

Ingredients:

- 8 ounces of turkey or chicken kielbasa sausage

- 2 cups of reduced-sodium chicken broth

- 2 cloves of garlic, minced

- 1 teaspoon of dried oregano

- 1 tablespoon of olive oil

- 1(15 ounces.) can of cannellini beans, drained and rinsed

- 6 cup of baby spinach leaves

- Pepper, to taste

Instructions:

1. Use non-stick cooking spray to spray a medium skillet. Cook the sausage and the juices are drained. Split into 1⁄4-1⁄2-inch rounds, and set aside.

2. In a big pot, add in the chicken broth and garlic cloves Place and bring to a boil on medium-high heat.

3. Add the oil, oregano, cooked sausage, and beans. Heat the beans until they are tender.

4. Once the leaves are wilted, add the spinach and cook. Stir and sprinkle on top with pepper.

5. Low Carb Cauliflower Pizza Crust Recipe (Crispy + 3 Ingredients)

(Ready in 45 Minutes, Serve 8, Difficulty: Normal)

Nutrition per Serving:

Calories 106, Protein: 10 g, Carbohydrates 5 g, Net Carbs 3 g, Fat 6 g, Fiber 2 g, Sugar 2 g.

Ingredients:

- 1 226 grams of cauliflower (florets only-about one large head)

- 1 1/2 cup of grated parmesan cheese

- 1 large egg

- 1/2 tablespoon of Italian seasoning (Optional)

- 1/2 teaspoon of garlic powder (optional)

Instructions:

1. The oven should be preheated to 400 degrees Fahrenheit (204 degrees Celsius). If you plan on using

a pizza stone (recommended) or a pizza pan, place a piece of parchment paper on a pizza peel.

2. In a food processor, blend the cauliflower florets until they are the consistency of rice.

3. Stir fry the cauliflower for about 10 minutes in a sauté pan on the stove, until the cauliflower is very soft. (This is important! If it's still crisp, the texture is off, so keep cooking until nice and soft.)

4. Meanwhile, whisk the egg in a large bowl. Stir in the cheese with parmesan cheese. Stir those in as well when using Italian seasoning and garlic powder.

5. When the cauliflower rice is thoroughly cooked and soft.

Option 1(more effort-recommended if making one large pizza): Place the cauliflower rice into a kitchen towel and squeeze over the sink.

Option 2(easier-better for making 2 smaller pizzas): Stir the cauliflower rice directly into the egg/cheese mixture.

With both options, make sure it's mixed very well. You may need to press with a spatula.

1. Spread the "dough" with your hands on the parchment paper, to about 1/4" thick. Depending on which option you chose in the previous step, you can make one large pizza or 2 smaller pizzas."

2. Use the pizza peel to transfer the parchment paper to the stone in the oven when using a pizza stone (recommended for best results). Otherwise, place the pan in the oven. Bake for about 20 minutes, until the top is dry and firm and the edges are a little golden.

Serving size: 1 slice of a large pizza, 2 slices of 2 smaller pizzas, or 1/8 of the entire recipe.

6. Creamy Pumpkin Soup

(Ready in 15 Minutes, Serve 4, Difficulty: Easy)

Nutrition per Serving:

Calories 162, Protein 5 g, Carbohydrates 18 g, Fat 9 g, Sodium 987mg, Potassium 373mg, Fiber 5 g, Sugar 7 g.

Ingredients:

- 2 cups of pumpkin puree

- 1 1/4 cup of vegetable broth

- 1 cup of reduced-fat coconut milk

- 1 small yellow onion

- 1 tablespoon of minced garlic

- 1 teaspoon of thyme

- 1/2 teaspoon of salt

- 1/4 teaspoon of pepper

- 4 tablespoon of pumpkin seeds

Instructions:

1. Chop the onion and garlic and sauté with 1/4 cup of vegetable stock in a medium saucepan.

2. To make a saucepan, add pumpkin puree, 1 cup of vegetable broth, coconut milk, thyme, salt, and pepper. To combine the ingredients, stir. Heat for 5 minutes, or until heated through on medium heat.

3. Transfer the soup to the blender and mix until all the ingredients are mixed.

4. Pour 4 bowls in. Use pumpkin seeds and black pepper to sprinkle.

Chapter 5: Soups Recipes

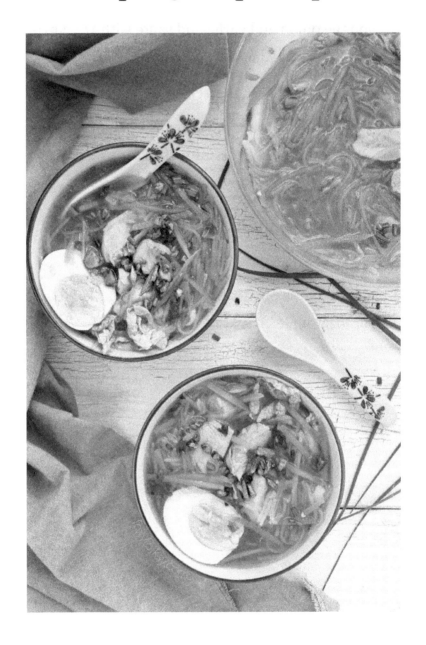

In this chapter, we are going to give you some delicious and mouthwatering recipes on Octavia Soups recipes.

1. Chicken Sotanghon

(Ready in 1 Hour and 45 Minutes, Serve 10, Difficulty: Easy)

Nutrition per Serving:

Calories 210, Protein 8.9 g, Carbohydrates 24.2 g, Fat 8.4 g, Cholesterol 29.8mg, Sodium 736.8mg.

Ingredients:

- 2 ½ cups of water

- 1 teaspoon of salt

- 453 g of chicken legs

- 1-ounce of dried shiitake mushrooms

- 8 ounces of bean thread noodles (cellophane noodles)

- 3 tablespoons of olive oil

- 1 onion, chopped

- 2 cloves of garlic, minced

- 1 ½ teaspoon of achiote powder

- 1 tablespoon of fish sauce

- Salt and pepper, to taste

- 2(14.5 ounces) cans of chicken broth

- Green onions, chopped

Instructions:

1. Bring 2 cups of water to a boil in a pot with one teaspoon of salt, cook the chicken in the boiling water until the middle is no longer pink and the juices are transparent, for about 10 minutes. A center-inserted instant-read thermometer can read at least 165 degrees F (74 degrees Celsius). Reserve the liquid, remove the chicken and cook until the meat is separated from the bones and two forks are shredded. Discard the bones and skin.

2. Allow soaking until pliable, around 30 minutes, while the chicken cools, put the shiitake mushrooms in

a bowl and pour enough warm water over them to fully cover. Remove and slice from the water and set aside. Place the bean thread noodles in the water and if needed, add more warm water to cover. Allow soaking for about 10 minutes until tender. Drain. If needed, cut the noodles.

3. Heat the olive oil over medium heat in a pan, cook and stir until the onion and garlic are tender about 5 minutes. Add the achiote powder and begin boiling and stirring until the red-orange color is well covered with the mixture. Stir in the mixture of shredded chicken meat, sliced shiitake mushrooms, fish sauce, and season to taste with salt and pepper.

4. Cook the mixture for about 5 minutes before adding the reserved liquid from the frying of the chicken and the chicken broth. Bring it to a 5-minute boil. Add the noodles and cook for an extra 5 minutes. Garnish with the green onion that will be eaten.

2. Southwestern Turkey Soup

(Ready in 45 Minutes, Serve 8, Difficulty: Normal)

Nutrition per Serving:

Calories 218, Protein 13.5 g, Carbohydrates 11.9 g, Fat 9.8 g, Cholesterol 32.5mg, Sodium 632mg.

Ingredients:

- 1 ½ cups of shredded cooked turkey

- 4 cups of vegetable broth

- 1(28 ounces) can of whole peeled tomatoes

- 1(4 ounces) can of chopped green Chile peppers

- 2 Roman (plum) tomatoes, chopped

- 1 onion, chopped

- 2 cloves of garlic, crushed

- 1 tablespoon of lime juice

- ½ teaspoon of cayenne pepper

- ½ teaspoon of ground cumin

- Salt and pepper, to taste

- 1 avocado, peeled, pitted, and diced

- ½ teaspoon of dried cilantro

- 1 cup of shredded Monterey Jack cheese.

Instructions:

1. Combine the turkey, broth, dried tomatoes, fresh tomatoes, green chilies, ginger, garlic, and lime juice in a large pot over medium heat. Use cayenne, cinnamon, and pepper to season. Bring it to a boil, reduce the flame, and simmer for 15 to 20 minutes.

2. Add the cilantro and avocado and boil for 15 to 20 minutes, until lightly thickened. Spoon into bowls for cooking, then finish with melted cheese.

3. Quick and Easy Chicken Noodle Soup

(Ready in 30 Minutes, Serve 6, Difficulty: Easy)

Nutrition per Serving:

Calories 216, Protein 13.4 g, Carbohydrates 12.1 g, Fat 6.1 g Cholesterol 46.4mg, Sodium 1356.8mg.

Ingredients:

- 1 tablespoon of butter

- ½ cup of chopped onion

- ½ cup of chopped celery

- 4(14.5 ounces) cans of chicken broth

- 1(14.5 ounces) can of vegetable broth

- 226 g of chopped cooked chicken breast

- 1 ½ cup of egg noodles

- 1 cup of sliced carrots

- ½ teaspoon of dried basil

- ½ teaspoon of dried oregano

- Salt and pepper, to taste

Instructions:

1. Melt the butter in a big pot over medium heat. Cook the onion and celery in the butter for 5 minutes, until just tender. Pour in the broths of meat and vegetables and stir in the chicken, carrots, noodles, basil, salt, pepper, and oregano.

2. Bring to a boil and simmer for 20 minutes before serving, then reduce the heat.

4. Chicken Tortilla Soup I

(Ready in 40 Minutes, Serve 8, Difficulty: Normal)

Nutrition per Serving:

Calories 377, Protein 23.1 g, Carbohydrates 30.9 g, Fat 19.1 g, Cholesterol 46.1mg, Sodium 943.2mg.

Ingredients:

- 1 onion, chopped

- 3 cloves of garlic, minced

- 1 tablespoon of olive oil

- 2 teaspoons of chili powder

- 1 teaspoon of dried oregano

- 1(28 ounces) can of crushed tomatoes

- 1(10.5 ounces) can of condensed chicken broth

- 1 ¼ cup of water

- 1 cup of whole corn kernels, cooked

- 1 cup of white hominy

- 1(4 ounces) can of chopped green Chile peppers

- 1(15 ounces) can of black beans, rinsed and drained

- ¼ cup of chopped fresh cilantro

- 2 boneless chicken breast halves, cooked and cut into bite-sized pieces

- Crushed tortilla chips

- 1 avocado, sliced

- Shredded Monterey jack cheese

- Green onions, chopped

Instructions:

1. Heat oil over low heat in a medium-sized stockpot. Cook the garlic and onion in the oil until tender.

2. Stir in the chili powder, onions, oregano, broth, and water. Bring it to a boil and let it simmer for 5-10 minutes.

3. Stir in the corn, chilies, beans, chicken, and cilantro. Simmer for 10 minutes.

4. Cover with crushed tortilla chips, avocado strips, cheese, and sliced green onion. Ladle soup into separate serving cups.

5. Egg Drop Soup

(Ready in 20 Minutes, Serve 6, Difficulty: Easy)

Nutrition per Serving:

Calories 211, Protein 7.5 g, Carbohydrates 4.8 g, Fat 6.7 g, Cholesterol 191mg, Sodium 1395.7mg.

Ingredients:

- 1 cup of chicken broth

- ¼ teaspoon of soy sauce

- ¼ teaspoon of sesame oil

- 1 teaspoon of cornstarch (Optional)

- 2 teaspoons of water (Optional)

- 1 egg, beaten

- 1 drop of yellow food coloring (Optional)

- 1 teaspoon of chopped fresh chives

- ⅛ teaspoon of salt (Optional)

- ½ teaspoon of ground white pepper (Optional)

Instructions:

1. Combine the chicken broth, soy sauce, and sesame oil in a small saucepan. Bring it to a boil. To dissolve the cornstarch, stir the cornstarch and water together and pour into the boiling broth.

2. If used, whisk gently before mixing in the egg and yellow food coloring. Before eating, season it with chives, salt, and pepper.

6. Cheeseburger Soup I

(Ready in 50 Minutes, Serve 8, Difficulty: Normal)

Nutrition per Serving:

Calories 121, Protein 18.9 g, Carbohydrates 18.6 g, Fat 18.3 g, Cholesterol 80.9mg, Sodium 595.6mg.

Ingredients:

- 226 g of ground beef

- ¾ cup of chopped onion

- ¾ cup of shredded carrots

- ¾ cup of chopped celery

- 1 teaspoon of dried basil

- 1 teaspoon of dried parsley

- 4 tablespoons of butter

- 3 cups of chicken broth

- 4 cups of cubed potatoes

- ¼ cup of all-purpose flour

- 2 cups of cubed Cheddar cheese

- 1 ½ cup of milk

- ¼ cup of sour cream

Instructions:

1. In a large pot, melt one tablespoon butter or margarine over medium heat: cook and stir vegetables and beef until beef is brown.

2. Stir in basil and parsley. Add broth and potatoes. Bring to a boil, then simmer until potatoes are tender, about 10-12 minutes.

3. Melt the remainder of butter and stir in flour. Add the milk, stirring until smooth.

4. Gradually add milk mixture to the soup, stirring constantly. Bring to a boil and reduce heat to simmer. Stir in cheese.

5. When cheese is melted, add sour cream and heat through. Do not boil.

Chapter 6: Vegan Recipes

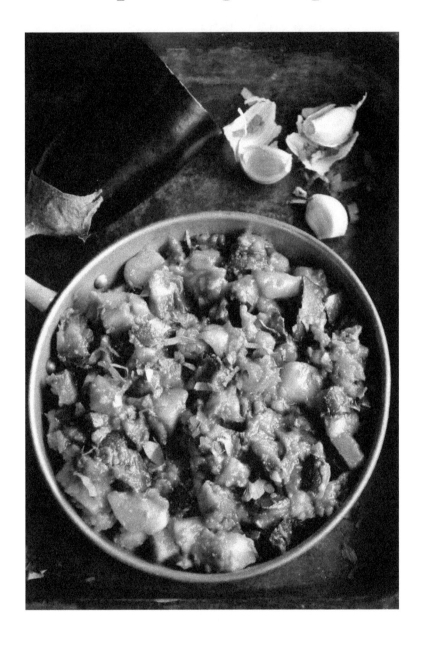

In this chapter we are going to give you some delicious and mouthwatering recipes on Octavia Vegan recipes.

1. Veggie Sweet Potato Burgers

(Ready in 35 Minutes, Serve 8, Difficulty: Normal)

Nutrition per Serving:

Calories 140, Protein 6.1 g, Carbohydrates 27.3 g, Fat 1.3 g, Cholesterol 0mg, Sodium 89mg.

Ingredients:

- 1 cup of cooked brown rice

- 1 cup of cooked black beans; no salt added

- 1 cup of cooked, mashed sweet potatoes

- ¼ cup of chopped roasted red bell peppers

- ¼ cup of diced tomatoes

- 3 green onions, finely chopped

- ¼ cup of shredded carrots

- ¼ cup of chopped cilantro

- 1 tablespoon of no-salt-added chili powder

- 2 cloves of garlic, minced

- 1 teaspoon of hot pepper sauce (such as Tabasco®)

- 1 teaspoon of ground cumin

Instructions:

1. The oven should be preheated to 400 degrees Fahrenheit (204 degrees Celsius). Line the parchment paper with a baking sheet.

2. In a large bowl, add the rice, beans, sweet potatoes, red bell peppers, tomatoes, green onions, cilantro, chili powder, carrots, garlic, spicy pepper sauce, and cumin. Place the mixture into 4 equal patties on the prepared baking sheet.

3. Bake for 15 minutes in the preheated oven. Flip the patties and bake until mildly crisp and browned about 15 more minutes.

2. Pasta

(Ready in 25 Minutes, Serve 3, Difficulty: Normal)

Nutrition per Serving:

Calories 218, Protein 8.5 g, Carbohydrates 34.7 g, Fat 2.3 g, Cholesterol 0mg, Sodium 438.9mg.

Ingredients:

- ⅓ cup of soy flour

- 1 cup of whole wheat flour

- ½ cup of spelt flour

- ¾ teaspoon of salt

- ½ cup of water, or as needed

Instructions:

1. Stir together the whole wheat flour, soy flour, spelled meal, and salt in a medium dish. Add water, and combine with the dough hook. To form a stiff yet pliable dough, use more water as needed. For about 10 minutes, mix or knead by hand. Cover, let the dough sit

for 30 minutes, or rest for at least an hour if you don't have a pasta machine.

2. Divide the dough into four parts, making things easier to roll. If you have one, pass the dough through a pasta machine or use a rolling pin to roll on a floured surface quite thinly, but not transparently.

3. Allow the pasta sheet to dry for a couple of minutes while you are making noodles. Flour dust, and roll into a loose channel. For linguine, or to the required size, slice the tube into 1/4-inch slices.

4. To cook: Put to a boil a big pot of lightly salted water. Add the pasta, then cook until al dente, depending on the thickness, for 1-5 minutes. Cooked pasta can float to the water's top.

3. Vegan Stuffed Peppers

(Ready in 55 Minutes, Serve 6, Difficulty: Normal)

Nutrition per Serving:

Calories 289, Protein 13.5 g, Carbohydrates 59.2 g, Fat 2 g, Cholesterol 0mg, Sodium 1982.3mg.

Ingredients:

- 4 red bell peppers, halved lengthwise and seeded

- 1 cup of water

- ½ cup of bulgur

- 1(24 ounces) of jar tomato sauce, or more to taste

- 2 cups of arugula

- 1 cup of corn kernels

- ½ cup of garbanzo beans, drained

- ½ cup of lima beans, drained

- ½ cup of black beans, rinsed and drained

- ½ cup of kidney beans, rinsed and drained

- 1 teaspoon of salt

- ½ teaspoon of paprika

- ½ teaspoon of dried basil

- ½ teaspoon of dried oregano

Instructions:

1. Preheat the oven to 350 degrees Fahrenheit (176 degrees Celsius). Line the aluminum foil with a 9x11-inch baking pan. In a baking pan, arrange the bell pepper halves.

2. In a shallow saucepan, put the water and the bulgur to a boil. Cover and cook for 12-15 minutes, until the bulgur is tender. Drain all extra water.

3. In a large dish, mix the bulgur, tomato sauce, arugula, corn, garbanzo beans, lima beans, black beans, kidney beans, cinnamon, paprika, basil, and oregano.

With a bulgur mixture, fill each bell pepper half generously.

4. Bake for 25-30 minutes in the preheated oven until bubbly and hot.

4. Quick Stuffed Tomatoes

(Ready in 55 Minutes, Serve 4, Difficulty: Normal)

Nutrition per Serving:

Calories 224, Protein 11.4 g, Carbohydrates 47.7 g, Fat 1.1 g, Cholesterol 1.3mg, Sodium 283.9mg.

Ingredients:

- 4 large tomatoes

- 1 ½ cups of vegetable broth

- ½ cup of heat-dried tomatoes, chopped

- 1 cup of couscous

- ¼ cup of shredded non-Fat mozzarella cheese

- ¼ cup of chopped fresh basil

- 2 tablespoons of minced fresh mint leaves

- ¼ teaspoon of ground black pepper

Instructions:

1. Preheat the oven to 375 degrees Fahrenheit (190 degrees Celsius).

2. Cut the fresh tomatoes in ½ crosswise and set aside to scoop out the pulp. To drain, invert the tomato shells onto paper towels.

3. Bring the broth and heat-dried tomatoes to boil in a small saucepan. Remove the heat from the saucepan and stir the couscous in. Cover to prepare for 5 minutes to stand.

4. Stir in the cheese, basil, pepper, and mint. Then stir in the tomato pulp gently.

5. In an 11x7 inch baking dish, put the tomato shells. Spoon the mixture of couscous into the shells, pressing the mixture into the shells tightly. Bake at 190 degrees Celsius (375 degrees F) for 25-30 minutes or until totally cooked.

5. Flavorful Rice

(Ready in 25 Minutes, Serve 8, Difficulty: Easy)

Nutrition per Serving:

Calories 231, Protein 6.1 g, Carbohydrates 60.5 g 2, Fat 4 g, Cholesterol 0mg, Sodium 81.9mg

Ingredients:

- 4 ½ cups of water

- 3 cups of uncooked white rice

- 2 tablespoons of olive oil

- 2 tablespoons of distilled white vinegar

- ½ teaspoon of dried basil

- ½ teaspoon of dried oregano

- 1 pinch of salt

- 1 pinch of ground black pepper

- 1(14.5 ounces) can of diced tomatoes, drained

Instructions:

1. Mix the sugar, flour, olive oil, vinegar, salt, pepper, basil, oregano, and tomatoes in your rice steamer. Cook in according to steamer settings.

6. Veggeroni

(Ready in 1 Hour and 20 Minutes, Serve 12, Difficulty: Hard)

Nutrition per Serving:

Calories 144, Protein 17.1 g, Carbohydrates 13.1 g, Fat 2.1 g, Cholesterol 0.1mg, Sodium 375.6mg.

Ingredients:

- 2 cups of wheat gluten

- ½ cup of isolated protein powder

- 1 tablespoon of agar-agar powder

- 1 ½ tablespoons of paprika

- 1 teaspoon of ground black pepper

- ½ teaspoon of red pepper flakes

- ½ teaspoon of cayenne pepper

- 1 tablespoon of fennel seed

- 2 teaspoons of garlic powder

- 1 envelope of dry onion soup mix

- 1 envelope of dry tomato soup mix

- 1 ½ cups of water

- 1 tablespoon of vegetable oil

- 1 teaspoon of liquid smoke flavoring

Instructions:

1. Preheat the oven to 325-degree Fahrenheit (165 degrees Celsius).

2. In a mixer, add gluten, protein powder, agar-agar, paprika, black pepper, red pepper, cayenne pepper, fennel seed, garlic powder, onion soup paste, and tomato soup. Grind the powder for 2-3 minutes, then pour it into a large mixing cup.

3. In the powdered mixture, stir the water, oil, and liquid smoke flavoring until moistened, knead the dough for 3-5 minutes. Shape the dough into a log of 2-3 inches, tightly wrap it in aluminum foil, and put it on a baking sheet.

4. Bake the Veggeroni for 1 hour in a preheated oven. Until slicing, cool absolutely.

Chapter 7: Meat Dishes

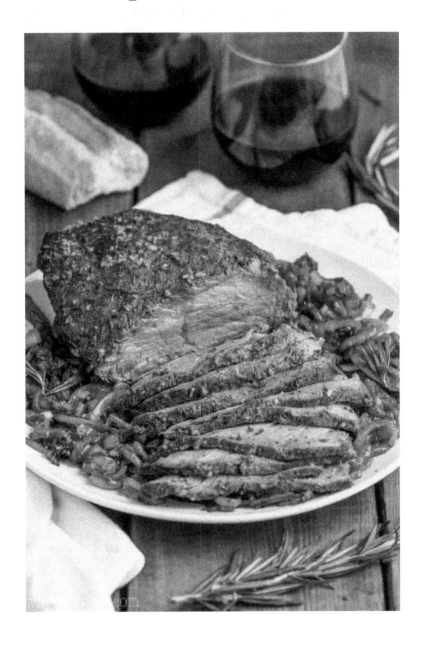

In this chapter, we are going to give you some delicious and mouthwatering recipes on Lean & Green Meat Dishes recipes.

1. Onion Meat Relish

(Ready in 35 Minutes, Serve 8, Difficulty: Normal)

Nutrition per Serving:

Calories 248, Protein 0.5 g, Carbohydrates 5.3 g, Fat 2.9 g, Cholesterol 7.6mg, Sodium 240.2mg.

Ingredients:

- 340 g of onion, cut into wedges and separated

- 2 tablespoons of butter

- 2 tablespoons of red wine vinegar

- ¼ tablespoon of salt

- ¼ teaspoon of ground black pepper

- 2 teaspoons of white sugar

Instructions:

1. Cook slowly in a medium saucepan over medium heat and stir in the onions and butter until the onions are tender, for about 10 minutes.

2. With the onions and butter, blend the red wine vinegar, ground black pepper, salt, and white sugar.

3. Continue to cook and stir until the mixture thickens, for about 10 minutes, to a chunky, spreadable consistency. Before serving, refrigerate.

2. Meat and Spinach Ravioli Filling

(Ready in 40 Minutes, Serve 15, Difficulty: Normal)

Nutrition per Serving:

Calories 107, Protein 6.5 g, Carbohydrates 1.6 g, Fat 8.2 g, Cholesterol 32.8mg, Sodium 124.1mg.

Ingredients:

- 453 g of ground beef

- 1 ½ cups of fresh spinach

- 5 tablespoons of grated Parmesan cheese

- 1 ¼ tablespoon of dried parsley

- ¼ cup of bread crumbs

- ¼ cup of olive oil

- 1 large egg

- ½ teaspoon of garlic salt

- 1 pinch of black pepper

Instructions:

1. Over medium-high prepare, heat a large skillet and stir in the ground beef. Cook and mix until the beef is crumbly, browned uniformly, and not pink anymore.

2. Drain some extra grease and dump it. Stir in the spinach and simmer for around 1-2 minutes, until wilted. Remove from the heat and allow 10 minutes to cool.

3. To a tub, pass the beef mixture. Combine the parmesan cheese, parsley, bread crumbs, egg, garlic salt, olive oil, and pepper and blend well. Run the filling until smooth, via a grinder (or puree in a food processor until smooth).

4. The filling can be stored for up to four days in the refrigerator or up to three months in the freezer.

3. Five Meat Habanero Chili

(Ready in 3 Hours and 5 Minutes, Serve 12, and Difficulty: Hard)

Nutrition per Serving:

Calories 309, Protein 26.7 g, Carbohydrates 26.4 g, Fat 21.3 g, Cholesterol 75.9mg, Sodium 1343.8mg.

Ingredients:

- 4 slices of hickory-smoked bacon

- 340 g of ground beef

- 453 g of bulk pork sausage

- 340 g of cubed beef stew meat

- 1 ½ cups of chopped onion

- 2 cloves of garlic, minced

- 1 stalk of celery, chopped

- ½ habanero pepper, seeded and minced, or to taste

- ½ large green bell pepper, chopped

- ½ large red bell pepper, chopped

- 1(28 ounces) can of tomato sauce

- 1 ½ teaspoon of ground cumin

- 2 cups of cubed cooked chicken

- 3(14.5 ounces) cans of fire-roasted diced tomatoes, with juice

- 1(15 ounces) can of cannellini beans, rinsed and drained

- 1(15 ounces) can of pinto beans, rinsed and drained

- 1(15 ounces) can of butter beans, rinsed and drained

- Salt and pepper, to taste

- ¾ cup of sour cream (Optional)

Instructions:

1. Place the bacon in a large pot and cook over medium-high heat for around 10 minutes, stirring periodically, until evenly browned.

2. Drain the bacon slices on a pan that is lined with paper towels. Stir in the ground beef, bacon, and beef stew meat in the same pot. Cook and mix until crumbly, uniformly browned, and no longer yellow, with the ground beef. Drain and set the meat in a bowl aside. Discard any excess grease.

3. Reduce heat to mild, then stir in the same big pot the onion, garlic, habanero pepper, celery, green bell pepper, and red bell pepper, cook and stir until smooth and translucent, around 5 minutes. Stir in the tomato sauce, then add the mixture of steak, sausage, bacon, and chicken. Stir in the sliced onions, pinto beans, cannellini beans, and butter beans. With salt and pepper, season. Over high heat, bring to a boil, reduce heat to low, and simmer for 2 hours. And use a dollop of sour cream to serve.

4. Kathy's Meat Hot Sauce

(Ready in 1 Hour and 10 Minutes, Serve 24, Difficulty: Normal)

Nutrition per Serving:

Calories 176, Protein 6.7 g, Carbohydrates 1.7 g, Fat 4.6 g, Cholesterol 22.9mg, Sodium 177mg.

Ingredients:

- 907 g of ground beef

- 2 ½ cups of tomato juice

- 1 ½ tablespoon of yellow mustard

- 1 tablespoon of ground black pepper

- 20 dashes of hot pepper sauce (such as Tabasco®)

- 5 teaspoons of chili powder

- 2 teaspoons of red pepper flakes

- ½ teaspoon of salt

Instructions:

1. In a large skillet, cook ground beef over medium heat for about 10 minutes until the meat is crumbly and no longer yellow; remove the excess Fat and move the ground beef to a large saucepan.

2. Mix in the beef with tomato paste, yellow mustard, black pepper, sweet pepper sauce, chili powder, red pepper, and salt.

3. Bring the sauce to a boil, reduce the heat to medium, and cook for 1 hour, stirring regularly.

5. Shelby's Microwave Meat Loaf

(Ready in 45 Minutes, Serve 6, Difficulty: Normal)

Nutrition per Serving:

Calories 382, Protein 29.5 g, Carbohydrates 22.8 g, Fat 18.8 g, Cholesterol 147.6mg, Sodium 664.7mg.

Ingredients:

- 1(8 ounces) can of tomato sauce

- ¼ cup of brown sugar

- 1 teaspoon of prepared mustard

- 2 eggs, lightly beaten

- 1 onion, minced

- ¼ cup of minced green bell pepper

- ¼ teaspoon of garlic powder

- ½ cup of saltine cracker crumbs

- 1 teaspoon of salt

- ¼ teaspoon of ground black pepper

- 907 g of extra lean ground beef

Instructions:

1. Mix the tomato sauce, brown sugar, and mustard in a small bowl and stir until the brown sugar has dissolved.

2. Mix the eggs, chopped onion and garlic powder, green pepper, cracker crumbs, salt, and black pepper in a big mixing bowl, mix in the ground beef and half the tomato mixture sauce, and stir until the meatloaf is fully mixed.

3. In a 2-quart microwave-safe baking dish, put the meat mixture into it. Spread over the meatloaf with the remaining tomato sauce mixture.

4. Cook in the high setting microwave oven until set, the juices run transparent, and the meat inside is no longer pink, 10-15 minutes, depending on the microwave power. 165 degrees Fahrenheit (75 degrees Celsius) can be read by an instant meat thermometer inserted into the middle of the loaf. If the loaf is baked,

remove some fat from the dish and rest, uncovered, 10-15 minutes before serving.

6. Poochie Meat Cakes

(Ready in 2 Hrs. Serve 36, Difficulty: Hard)

Nutrition per Serving:

Calories 309, Protein 14.1 g, Carbohydrates 12.8 g, Fat 22.1 g, Cholesterol 64.3mg, Sodium 73mg.

Ingredients:

- 1 ½ cup of brown rice

- 3 cups of water

- 2 large potatoes, grated

- 4 large carrots, grated

- 2 large stalks of celery, chopped

- 3721 g of ground beef

- 8 eggs

- 1 dash of salt

- ¼ cup of olive oil

- 1 ½ cup of regular rolled oats

Instructions:

1. Preheat the oven to 400 degrees Fahrenheit (204 degrees Celsius). 36 cups in 3 big muffin tins are oiled.

2. Combine the rice in a medium saucepan with water. Cook for 10 minutes and bring to a boil over high pressure, uncovered. Lower the heat, cover it and simmer for 20 minutes. Remove from heat, cool for a few minutes, and then use a fork to fluff and set aside.

3. Combine the potatoes, onions, celery, ground beef, and eggs in a large dish. Using your hands or a strong spoon to blend the ingredients.

4. Mix well with salt, olive oil, rolled oats, and rice.

5. Fill some of the meat mixtures with each muffin cup, then pat it down to make it solid. Bake until the surface feels fixed, or 45 minutes. Cool it on a rack for 10 minutes or more.

6. By flipping the muffin tin upside down above an aluminum foil layer, remove the meat cakes. To release the cake, tap each muffin cup. Refrigerate or freeze in plastic bags that are sealed.

Chapter 8: Salad Recipes

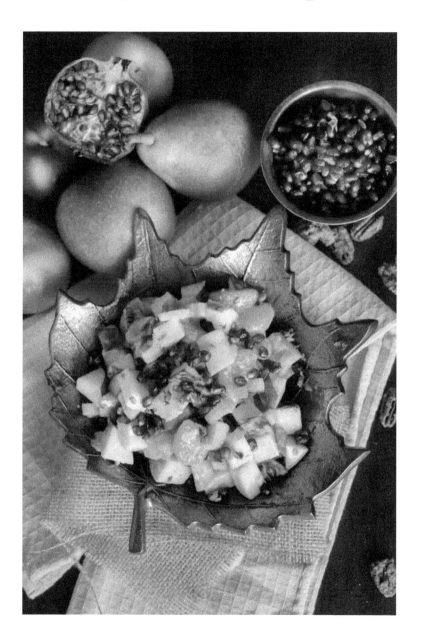

In this chapter we are going to give you some delicious and mouthwatering recipes on Lean & Green Salad recipes.

1. Autumn Waldorf Salad

(Ready in 40 Minutes, Serve 2, Difficulty: Normal)

Nutrition per Serving:

Calories 312, Protein 3.2 g, Carbohydrates 70.3 g, Fat 5.5 g, Cholesterol 0mg, Sodium 54.8mg.

Ingredients:

- ¼ cup of plain yogurt

- 1 ½ teaspoons of brown sugar

- 1 pear, diced

- 1 apple, diced

- 1 cup of sliced celery (Optional)

- ½ cup of raisins

- ¼ cup of dried cranberries

- 2 tablespoons of chopped walnuts

- 1 dash of ground cinnamon (optional)

- 1 dash of ground nutmeg (optional)

Instructions:

1. To make a dressing, blend the yogurt and brown sugar in a cup.

2. In a cup, blend the peach, apple, cranberries, celery, raisins, and walnuts.

3. To mix, add dressing and toss properly. Sprinkle the end with cinnamon and nutmeg.

4. Before serving, cool the salad for at least 30 minutes.

2. Hot Fruit Salad

(Ready in 40 Minutes, Serve 12, Difficulty: Normal)

Nutrition per Serving:

Calories 149, Protein 0.7 g, Carbohydrates 37.7 g, Fat 0.1 g, Cholesterol 0mg, Sodium 15.3mg.

Ingredients:

- 1(20 ounces) jar of chunky applesauce

- 1(21 ounces) can of cherry pie filling

- 1(15 ounces) can of sliced peaches, drained

- 1(11 ounces) can of mandarin orange segments, drained

- 1(8 ounces) can of pineapple chunks

- ½ cup of brown sugar

- 1 teaspoon of ground cinnamon

Instructions:

1. In a slow cooker, pour the applesauce, cherry pie filling, peaches diced, pineapple, mandarin oranges, brown sugar, and cinnamon.

2. On a low setting, cover and cook for 90 minutes.

3. Zesty Apple Salad

(Ready in 40 Minutes, Serve 4, Difficulty: Normal)

Nutrition per Serving:

Calories 236, Protein 4.4 g, Carbohydrates 49.3 g, Fat 3.4 g, Cholesterol 2.8mg, Sodium 67.2mg.

Ingredients:

- 2 Granny Smith apples, diced

- 1(15 ounces) can of mandarin oranges, drained

- 1 ½ cups of miniature marshmallows

- 1 cup of halved seedless red grapes

- 1(8 ounces) container of lemon yogurt

- 2 tablespoons of chopped walnuts

Instructions:

1. In a bowl, combine the strawberries, bananas, grapes, yogurt, marshmallows, and walnuts.

4. Really, Truly Gorgeous Dried Fruit Salad

(Ready in 40 Minutes, Serve 12, Difficulty: Normal)

Nutrition per Serving:

Calories 211, Protein 2.7 g, Carbohydrates 51.6 g, Fat 1.9 g, Cholesterol 0mg, Sodium 9mg.

Ingredients:

- 8 ounces of dried figs

- 8 ounces of dried apricots

- 8 ounces of pitted prunes

- ½ cup of dried cranberries

- ½ cup of raisins

- ½ cup of golden raisins

- ¼ cup of pine nuts

- 1 tablespoon of honey

Instructions:

1. In a cup, mix the figs, apricots, raisins, prunes, cranberries, and golden raisins. Only dump enough water in to cover it. Cover the bowl and soak for at least 8 hours overnight.

2. Pour the fruits into a saucepan with the soaking water. Stir in the honey and pine nuts.

3. Bring to a boil, roast, stirring regularly, around 30 minutes, until the fruit is tender but still retains its form. Remove the fruit and liquid from the heat and add it to the cup, taking care not to split the fruit. Cool to room temperature.

5. Pomegranate Ambrosia Salad

(Ready in 40 Minutes, Serve 12, Difficulty: Normal)

Nutrition per Serving:

Calories 167, Protein 1.5 g, Carbohydrates 27.1 g, Fat 7.3 g, Cholesterol 2.1mg, Sodium 41.4mg.

Ingredients:

- 2 cups of pomegranate seeds

- 1(15 ounces) can of pineapple tidbits, drained

- 4 bananas, peeled and sliced

- 3 cups of peeled, cored, and chopped tart apple

- ½ cup of chopped pecans

- 3 tablespoons of mayonnaise

- 2 tablespoons of creamy salad dressing, e.g., Miracle Whip ™

Instructions:

1. Combine the pomegranate seeds, bananas, pineapple, apples, and pecans in a large dish. Stir in the sauce with mayonnaise and lettuce until finely coated.

2. Before serving, cover and refrigerate overnight.

6. Autumn Salad with Caramel-Sesame Dressing

(Ready in 40 Minutes, Serve 1, Difficulty: Normal)

Nutrition per Serving:

Calories 223, Protein 4.5 g, Carbohydrates 52 g, Fat 2.6 g, Cholesterol 0.2mg, Sodium 140.1mg.

Ingredients:

- 1 ½ cup of chopped fresh spinach

- 1 ½ cup of chopped romaine lettuce

- ½ ripe Bartlett pear, skinned, cored, and diced into medium chunks

- ½ Fuji apple, skin on, cored, and diced into medium chunks

- ¼ cup of halved seedless red grapes (Optional)

- 3 tablespoons of rice vinegar

- 1 tablespoon of caramel topping, such as Hershey's®

- ¼ teaspoon of sesame oil

- ¼ teaspoon of toasted sesame seeds

Instructions:

1. Place on a plate of spinach, pear, romaine lettuce, apple, and grapes.

2. In a bowl, combine the vinegar, sesame oil, caramel topping, and sesame seeds.

3. Pour the salad over the dressing.

Chapter 9: Dessert Recipes

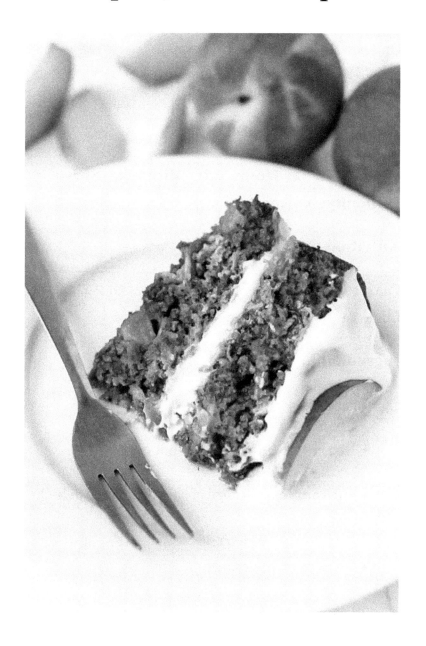

In this chapter, we are going to give you some delicious and mouthwatering recipes

On Lean & Green Dessert recipes.

1. Applesauce Salad

(Ready in 1 Hour, 20 Minutes, Serve 8, Difficulty: Normal)

Nutrition per Serving:

Calories 155, Protein 2 g, Carbohydrates 38.2 g, Fat 0 g, Cholesterol 0mg, Sodium 103.5mg.

Ingredients:

- 2 cups of water

- ½ cup of cinnamon red-hot candies

- 1(6 ounces) package of cherry flavored Jell-O® Mix

- 2 cups of applesauce

Instructions:

1. Put it to a boil with water. Dissolve the red-hot sweets in the boiling water with the cinnamon.

2. Add in and heat the cherry-flavored gelatin.

3. Transfer to a medium tub. With a mix of applesauce. Freeze in the refrigerator for 4 hours or until completely gelled.

2. Banana in Caramel Sauce

(Ready in 20 Minutes, Serve 2, Difficulty: Normal)

Nutrition per Serving:

Calories 258, Protein 3.1 g, Carbohydrates 79 g, Fat 50.9 g, Cholesterol 162.9mg, Sodium 193.4mg.

Ingredients:

- ½ cup of butter

- 1 cup of superfine sugar

- 1 ¼ cup of heavy cream

- 4 medium (7" to 7-7/8" long) bananas, peeled and halved lengthwise

Instructions:

1. Melt butter over medium heat in a large, heavy skillet. Stir in the sugar and boil, stirring well until the sugar is molten and slightly brown. Gently stir in the milk (mixture will bubble up).

2. Let the mixture cook for 1 minute, then bring it to medium heat. Place the bananas in the pan and cook until hot, for around 2 minutes. Serve warm.

3. Ice Cream Sandwich Cake

(Ready in 30 Minutes, Serve 12, Difficulty: Normal)

Nutrition per Serving:

Calories 278, Protein 6.5 g, Carbohydrates 85.4 g, Fat 24.8 g, Cholesterol 39.8mg, Sodium 260mg

Ingredients:

- 24 vanilla ice cream sandwiches, unwrapped

- 2(8 ounces) containers of whipped topping (such as Cool Whip®), thawed

- 1(12 ounces) jar of hot fudge ice cream topping, warmed

- 1(12 ounces) jar of caramel ice cream topping

- ¼ cup of chopped pecans, or to taste

Instructions:

1. Arrange a line of ice cream sandwiches on top of a layer of whipped topping, hot fudge topping, and caramel topping at the bottom of a 9x13-inch dish. Repeat layering, whipped topping, hot fudge topping, and caramel topping for the leftover ice cream sandwiches, finishing with a top layer of whipped topping.

2. Sprinkle pecans. Cover the dish with aluminum foil and freeze for a minimum of 30 minutes until set.

4. Virginia Apple Pudding

(Ready in 40 Minutes, Serve 6, Difficulty: Normal)

Nutrition per Serving:

Calories 384, Protein 3.8 g, Carbohydrates 57.5 g, Fat 16.4 g, Cholesterol 43.9mg, Sodium 343.3mg.

Ingredients:

- ½ cup of butter, melted

- 1 cup of white sugar

- 1 cup of all-purpose flour

- 2 teaspoons of baking powder

- ¼ teaspoon of salt

- 1 cup of milk

- 2 cups of chopped, peeled apple

- 1 teaspoon of ground cinnamon

Instructions:

1. Preheat the oven to 375 degrees Fahrenheit (190 degrees Celsius).

2. Combine the butter, sugar, flour, baking powder, salt, and milk in a shallow baking dish until smooth.

3. Combine the apples and cinnamon in a microwave-proof dish. Microwave, 2-5 minutes, until the apples are tender. Onto the middle of the batter, dump the apples.

4. Bake for 30 minutes, or until crispy, in a preheated oven.

Conclusion

Healthy eating provides many health benefits to people. The importance of including vegetables and lean proteins in the daily diet is well known. This, together with a low carbohydrate intake, will accelerate weight loss and metabolism among those who follow this type of diet. This is the principle that governs the Lean and Green diet, which is a balanced diet to help you lose weight and keep it off. The Lean and Green diet focuses on the consumption of lean proteins and green vegetables, which bring multiple benefits to the body, in addition to reducing carbohydrate intake, which allows you to burn stored fat and accelerate metabolism.

In general, it is a hypocaloric and low-carbohydrate diet and focuses on the intake of proteins from poultry meats such as chicken, turkey, fish or eggs, and some non-starchy vegetables, limiting, or excluding foods such as grains, legumes, breads, sweets, noodles and starchy vegetables, some nuts and seeds. Additionally, sugary drinks, alcohol, refined cereals and fried foods should be avoided.

It should be noted that if you want to start with an eating plan, it is important to consult with a doctor or health professional, especially if you have any special condition such as being pregnant, breastfeeding or if you have any disease, such as diabetes or heart disease.

CPSIA information can be obtained
at www.ICGtesting.com
Printed in the USA
BVHW041516190321
602997BV00010B/570